I0115478

All About
MULTIPLE SCLEROSIS

By Laura Flynn R.N., B.N., M.B.A., in consultation with her nurse educator associates and physicians who assisted in contributing and editing.

ISBN No: 978 1 896616 79 7

© 2011, 2017 Mediscript Communications Inc.

The publisher, Mediscript Communications Inc., acknowledges the financial support of the Government of Canada through the Canadian Book Fund for our publishing activities.

Printed in Canada

www.mediscript.net

Book and Front Cover design by:
Brian Adamson, www.AdamsonGraphics.net

MS1002010

ALL ABOUT BOOKS
Trusted • Reliable • Certified

- 40+ titles available
- Comply with accreditation and regulatory bodies
- Suitable for caregivers, boomers with elderly parents, health workers, auxiliary health staff & patients
- Self study style with "test yourself" section
- Health On the Net (HON) certified

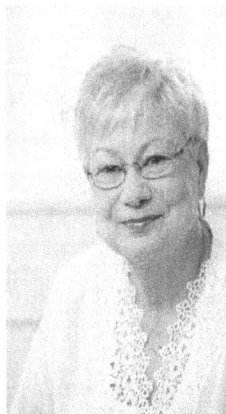

Some of our titles:

Alzheimers Disease	Arthritis	Multiple Sclerosis
Pain	Strokes	Elder Abuse
Falls Prevention	Incontinence	Nutrition & Aging
Personal Care	Positioning	Confusion
Transferring people	Care of the Back	Skin Care

For complete list of titles go to www.mediscript.net

Contact: 1 800 773 5088
Fax 1800 639 3186 • Email: mediscript30@yahoo.ca

CONTENTS

Introduction 4

Message from the publisher 6

Have you heard 7

How much do you know 8

CORE CONTENT

What is Multiple Sclerosis? 13

How common is MS? 15

Risk factors 16

Signs and symptoms 18

How to diagnose the disease 21

Diagnostic tests for MS 23

Treatment 24

Safety issues 29

Care considerations for healthcare workers 31

Case example 37

Conclusion 41

Check your knowledge 42

Test yourself 43

References 47

INTRODUCTION

This book provides basic, non controversial and trusted information that can help a wide spectrum of readers.

The primary objective of the information is to help a person provide effective quality care to a loved one or someone in his or her care.

After reading this material you will have an overview of Multiple Sclerosis (MS) and greater understanding of how to provide quality care to people with the disease.

All the information is reliable and was written by a group of eminent nurse educators who ensured the information complies with best practice guidelines and satisfies the various accreditation and regulatory bodies. Because there is so much unreliable information on the internet, you can be assured the "All About" publications are HON (Health On the Net) certified.

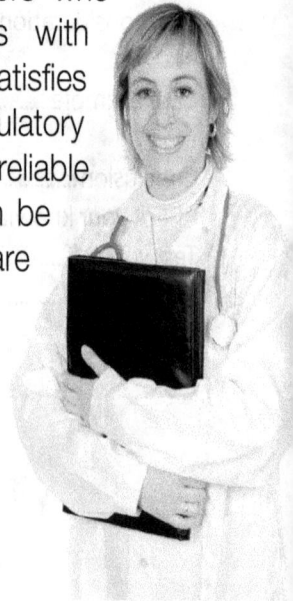

This book can be an invaluable aid to:

- A caregiver caring for a relative or friend;

- A health worker seeking a reference aid;

- A person with MS and her family;

- Any person involved in health care wishing to expand his or her knowledge.

SOMETHING TO THINK ABOUT...

Life is no brief candle to me.
It is a sort of splendid torch
that I have got hold of
for the moment,
and I want to make it burn
as brightly as possible
before handing it on to
future generations.

George Bernard Shaw

AN IMPORTANT MESSAGE
FROM THE PUBLISHER

Each person's treatment, advice, medical aids, physical therapy and other approaches to health care are unique and highly dependant upon the diagnosis and overall assessment by the medical team.

We emphasize therefore that the information within this book is not a substitute for the advice and treatment from a health care professional.

This book provides generic information concerning the issues around MS and common sense, well-established care practices for people with this condition and their families.

With all this in mind, the publishers and authors disclaim any responsibility for any adverse effects resulting directly or indirectly from the suggestions contained within this book or from any misunderstanding of the content on the part of the reader.

The following are actual classified ads that appeared in newspapers:

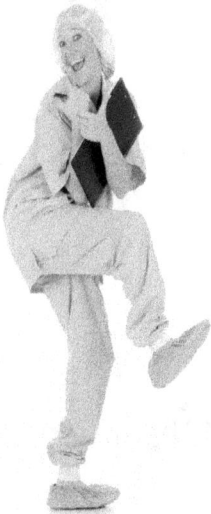

- Washer $100. Owned by clean bachelor who seldom washed.

- Snow Blower for sale. Only used on snowy days.

- 83 Toyota Hunchback - $2000

- **FREE:** 1 can of pork and beans with purchase of 3 BR 2 BATH Home.

Source: www.funnymail.com

HOW MUCH DO YOU KNOW

It helps to figure out how much you know before starting. In this way you will have an idea as to the gaps in your knowledge prior to reading the content. Please circle to indicate the best answer. Remember, at this stage, you are not expected to know all the answers:

1. Multiple Sclerosis (MS) is a chronic disease that affects the brain and spinal cord.

a True

b False

2. As many as 80% of people with MS have a relative with the disease.

a True

b False

3. MS affects very few people.

a True

b False

4. Most people who get MS are 60 years of age or older.

a True

b False

5. Canada has one of the lowest rates of MS in the world.

a True

b False

6. Some people with MS state that their greatest problem from the disease is:

a Overwhelming fatigue

b Itchiness as a side effect of the disease

c Not being able to get to sleep at night

d Waking up often during the night

7. One of the factors that seem to make it more likely that someone will get MS is:

a Following a diet that includes few dairy products

b Following a diet that includes lots of high caffeine foods and drinks

c Being exposed to certain viruses

d Living in a tropical climate

NOTES ON ANSWERS

ANSWERS

1. a. True. Multiple Sclerosis is a chronic disease that affects the brain and spinal cord.

2. b. False. Approximately 20% of MS people have a relative with the disease.

3. b. False. The disease affects over 2.5 million people throughout the world.

4. b. False. It usually strikes people between the ages of 20 and 40.

5. b. False. Canadians have one of the highest rates of MS in the world.

6. a. People with MS sometimes feel so tired that they cannot perform their normal daily activities.

7. c. Being exposed to certain common viruses may increase the risk of getting MS in some people.

WHAT IS MULTIPLE SCLEROSIS?

Multiple Sclerosis is a chronic disease that affects the brain and spinal cord. The brain and spinal cord make up the central nervous system. MS is a disease that usually, but not always, results in permanent disability.

In the central nervous system, a substance called myelin covers the nerves. Myelin protects the nerves. It also helps to send messages between the brain and spinal cord and other parts of the body. In MS, inflammation damages the myelin. Over time, the nerves become damaged as well. This damage causes many areas of scarring called sclerosis. These scars slow down or block the ability of the nerves to send messages. Since the central nervous system controls body functions and sensations, people with MS can have many different problems. These problems include difficulty walking or speaking, vision disturbances, and numbness or tingling of the arms and legs.

There are several types of MS. These include:

Benign. Symptoms of this type are fairly mild. They do not get worse and they do not lead to permanent disability. This type of MS is found in 10-15% of people who have been diagnosed with the disease.

Relapsing-remitting type causes a sudden outbreak of symptoms that occurs every one to three years. The symptoms last for a few weeks or months and then slowly go away. Symptoms may not appear again for years. However, they may get worse each time they return. About 85% of persons with MS have this type at the time they are diagnosed.

Primary progressive MS causes rapid decline of the client's condition. After the symptoms first appear, the disease progresses steadily without periods of relief from symptoms (remission). About 15% to 20% of people with MS begin with this form of the disease.

Secondary progressive type of MS is a stage of constant worsening (deterioration) of the client's condition. This type occurs after the client has had relapsing-remitting MS for a number of years.

Progressive relapsing is a rare type of MS. It occurs in less than five percent of people who have the disease. The client's condition worsens constantly. He/she also has sudden episodes of new symptoms or worsening of symptoms that already exist.

CONSIDER FOR A MOMENT ...

Are you currently caring for a person with MS?

If so, do you know what type of

MS the person has?

HOW COMMON IS MULTIPLE SCLEROSIS?

MS is the most common cause of disability affecting the brain and spinal cord in young adults. About half of MS patients are unable to walk without help 15 years after being diagnosed. However, about 70% of people with MS are able to continue to lead active, productive lives with the help of treatment.

The disease affects over 2.5 million people throughout the world. It is most common among people who live in northern climates, in cities (urban areas), and those who earn a fairly high income (higher socioeconomic groups). MS is twice as common in women than it is in men. It usually strikes people between the ages of 20 and 40.

MS is very common in North America. Canadians have one of the highest rates of MS in the world. Every day in Canada three more people are diagnosed with this disease. In the United States, MS affects as many as 350,000 people.

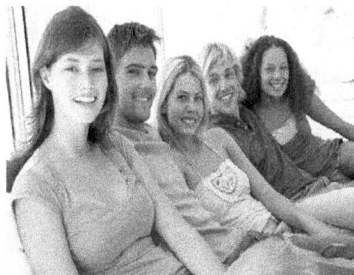

RISK FACTORS

The exact cause of MS is unknown. There is strong evidence that MS develops as a result of the body attacking and damaging its own myelin. This is called an autoimmune response. Under normal conditions, the immune cells help us to fight disease. But doctors believe that in MS, the immune cells mistakenly help to destroy the myelin that protects nerves. Exactly why the body damages its own myelin is not known.

Doctors believe that a number of risk factors may contribute to the development of MS. These risk factors include:

Heredity

MS seems to run in families. People who have a family member with MS have a greater chance of developing the disease. As many as 20% of people with MS have a relative with the disease.

Geography

Countries with temperate climates, such as those in North America, Northern Europe, Australia, and New Zealand, have a much higher rate of MS than tropical countries or climates.

Infection with certain viruses

Being exposed to certain common viruses may increase the risk of getting MS in some people. For example, many people with MS have been exposed to the Herpes simplex virus (causes fever blisters) or to conditions such as measles or rubella (also called German measles).

Diet

Research has shown that people at high risk for MS eat a diet high in animal fats and dairy products. MS is much less common in countries where people eat few dairy products.

Other factors may help to cause MS. These include trauma, poor nutrition, and anorexia nervosa (an eating disorder). Stress, overwork, fatigue, pregnancy, and acute infections of the breathing passages may occur before the onset of MS.

CONSIDER FOR A MOMENT ...

Are any of these risk
factors present in your life?

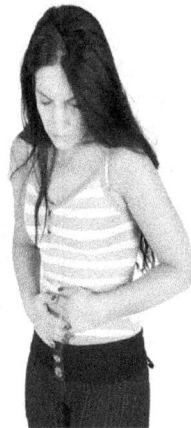

SIGNS AND SYMPTOMS

The first episode of signs and symptoms of MS may last for only a few hours or days. They may not show up again for weeks, months, or even years. Symptoms may change from day to day and be difficult for the person to describe. Also, other conditions can cause signs and symptoms similar to MS. Some of the conditions that can cause similar symptoms are stroke, diabetes, Lyme disease, tumors of the central nervous system, thyroid disease, chronic fatigue syndrome, and a lack of vitamin B12.

In most cases, vision problems or changes in sensation are the first signs that something might be wrong. The person may complain of blurred or double vision. A burning sensation, a feeling of tingling ("pins and needles"), or numbness in the arms or legs may occur.

Other common symptoms include the following:

Muscle problems

These include weakness, difficulty walking, loss of balance, difficulty coordinating movements, trembling, muscle spasms, and not being able to move arms or legs.

Bladder problems

The person may complain of having an urgent need to go the bathroom. Frequent visits to the bathroom may be needed. The person may not be able to control the need to pass urine (incontinent). Bladder infections are common.

Bowel problems

The person may complain of being constipated. He may not be able to control having bowel movements (incontinent).

Fatigue

The person may report feeling very, very tired. People sometimes feel so tired that they cannot perform their normal daily activities. This feeling of exhaustion can occur at any time of the day without warning.

Other symptoms include difficulty speaking or trouble swallowing. The person may be very irritable. Sometimes people have "mood swings." This means that they may be very depressed and sad and then suddenly, without reason, become very happy. People with MS are sometimes not able to control their emotions.

CONSIDER FOR A MOMENT ...

Have you cared for someone with

MS who has the signs and symptoms described above?

Were there any other symptoms not mentioned here?

HOW TO DIAGNOSE THE DISEASE

No single test can detect MS. It can take months or even years before a doctor is able to make a definite diagnosis of MS. People can become quite frustrated and upset trying to find a reason for symptoms that come and go without warning. Sometimes healthcare professionals believe that people are imagining their symptoms. They refer them to psychiatrists or psychologists. Listen carefully to what the people in your care tell you. A thorough client history may be the best indicator of MS.

Doctors often rely on the following guidelines to help them make a diagnosis of MS:

- The client's symptoms suggest damage to the nervous system in more than one place.

- The client's symptoms have gotten worse for more than six months.

- The client must have experienced symptoms on at least two separate occasions. These symptoms must have lasted for more than one day. The symptoms must disappear for at least one month before they reappear.

- Symptoms are caused by damage to the "white matter" of the central nervous system only.

- The client is between 10 and 50 years of age.

- The client does not have any disease or condition (such as a tumor or a stroke) that may cause similar symptoms.

Although no single test can definitely diagnosis MS, there are some tests that can help doctors to recognize the disease. In order to help the people in your care, you need to understand what these tests are and what they mean. The table on the following page explains these diagnostic tests.

DIAGNOSTIC TESTS FOR MS

DIAGNOSTIC TEST	EXPLANATION
Electroencephalography (EEG)	Electrodes are placed on the scalp and the EEG records the electrical activity of the brain. The test does not cause any pain or discomfort. The night before the test, people are asked to wash their hair. They should not use any oils, hairsprays, or lotions on their hair before the test. People should not eat or drink anything with caffeine such as coffee, colas, tea, or chocolate since this will interfere with test results. About one-third of the people who have MS have abnormal EEGs.
Lumbar Puncture	During a lumbar puncture a needle is placed in the client's back, in the space next to the spinal cord. Fluid (called cerebrospinal fluid) is removed from that space and checked for abnormalities. The person usually lies on his/her side and must stay very still during the procedure. Medication to reduce pain is given before the lumbar puncture. However, the procedure can still cause some discomfort. In people with MS the cerebrospinal fluid has an abnormally high amount of white blood cells and other substances.
Evoked Potential Studies	These studies focus on changes and responses in brain activity that take place when certain senses on the body are stimulated. The person is told to shampoo his hair before the test. Electrodes are placed on his scalp. The person's responses to different kinds of stimuli, such as flashing lights and various noises, are tested. Nerve impulses transmit at a much slower rate than normal for about 80% of people with MS.

TREATMENT

There is no cure for MS. The goals of treatment are to: 1) shorten the length of time symptoms last, and 2) reduce, as much as possible, the damage done to the person's functioning as a result of severe reappearance of symptoms (exacerbations).

For some people, the signs and symptoms of MS are mild and do not occur very often. These people may only need to be observed. Some will benefit from counseling to learn how to deal with a chronic disease. In others, symptoms occur more often. The disease is more severe and debilitating. These people may need treatment to reduce the effects of the disease.

Medications

Until recently, the medications most often used to treat MS were ones called corticosteroids. Since myelin damage is caused by inflammation, these medications help by reducing the inflammation in nerve tissue. They also shorten the time the attacks last. However, if someone uses corticosteroids for a long time, side effects, such as acne, weight gain, and high blood pressure, might occur. Researchers are working on developing new drugs to help sufferers of MS. Recently, other types of medications have been used to help them.

Drugs for MS work in different ways. They may fight infections caused by viruses and regulate the immune system. They may work to stop the immune system's attack on myelin. Some medications help the muscles to relax. They control the muscle spasms that are so common in MS. Still other medications help to control fatigue.

These other types of drugs for MS may also have side effects. Some cause symptoms similar to the flu. Others cause flushing and shortness of breath after the medication is injected. Find out about the side effects of any medications that your client is taking.

Treating fatigue

Some people with MS say that overwhelming feelings of tiredness cause them the most problem. Some medications help reduce fatigue. As well, people with MS should avoid extreme physical activity. Mild to moderate exercise may, however, may help to lessen fatigue and to maintain functioning. People who suffer from MS should consult with their doctors about what type and how much exercise is good for them. As a caregiver, help them schedule rest periods throughout the day. Heat and humidity seem to make the fatigue worse.

Treating muscle problems

Muscle spasms cause either sustained stiffness or spasms that come and go, especially at night. Medications, stretching, range-of-motion exercises, and correct positioning help muscles relax and function well.

Other muscle problems include weakness, loss of balance, and difficulty coordinating movement. Physical therapy and assistive devices, such as canes and wheelchairs, may be helpful.

Treating bladder problems

Common bladder problems include incontinence, infections, and frequent urgent needs to go to the bathroom. A person with MS may have a problem storing urine in the bladder. He/she may not be able to fully empty the bladder. Some people have a combination of both problems.

Certain medications, vitamin C tablets, and cranberry juice may help prevent bladder problems. Catheterization is another treatment measure that is often used. With catheterization, the a catheter (drainage tube) is inserted into the bladder several times a day. The tube drains urine from the bladder. Some people may use an indwelling or Foley catheter. An indwelling catheter may be left in place for days or even weeks. It connects to a drainage bag. People need to drink an adequate amount of fluids to help avoid bladder infections.

Treating bowel problems

Adding fiber to the diet can help bowel problems such as incontinence and constipation. Good sources of fiber are fruits, vegetables, and whole grain breads and cereals. Certain medications also help to deal with constipation.

Treating sexual problems

People with MS may have sexual problems. Some men may not be able to attain an erection. Women may experience pain and dryness with intercourse. Some people may also complain of decreased sex drive and difficulty achieving orgasm.

Medications are available that may help improve the situation. Women may find use of a water-based lubricant helpful for them. Some men choose to have an implant inserted in their penis. This procedure helps them to have an erection. People having problems should consult with their physician. Honest discussion with their sexual partner about what does and does not help may also be helpful.

Treating depression

Dealing with MS and its signs and symptoms is not easy. Some people become depressed as they attempt to deal with this devastating disease. Stress may add to the severity of symptoms. Medications that treat depression or anxiety may help. Emotional counseling may also help to reduce depression.

The treatment team

Many healthcare professionals are involved in the treatment of MS clients. Nurses and doctors help treat MS clients. Speech/language pathologists assist clients who have difficulty speaking or swallowing. Physical therapists work with clients who experience muscle spasms, weakness, and difficulty walking and maintaining their balance. Occupational therapists help clients who need to learn new ways of bathing, dressing, working, and, in general, carrying out their normal activities of daily living. Therapeutic recreation specialists help clients plan and carry out fulfilling leisure activities that help them enjoy life and maintain functioning.

SAFETY ISSUES

Consider the signs and symptoms of MS – fatigue, muscle weakness, muscle spasms, blurred vision, loss of balance, and numbness in the arms and legs. These signs and symptoms make it more likely that accidents, such as falls or burns, can happen.

If you are caring for someone in her home, some issues for you to consider include:

- How difficult is it for her to use the stairs?

- Do loose rugs or thick carpet pose a hazard for trips?

- Is the house well lighted? Does she use a nightlight?

- Can she easily exit the home in an emergency?

- Are the floors cluttered with obstacles that could cause tripping?

- Are handrails present on the staircase and in other areas as needed?

- Does she take baths or showers? Is there anyone nearby to offer help as needed when your client does bathe?

- How does she manage cooking? Is she lifting heavy pots and saucepans off the stove?

The person with MS is often the best source of information. Find out what he or she thinks the safety issues are. Discuss ways to improve on safety.

CONSIDER FOR A MOMENT ...

Can you identify other safety issues
for the people in your care?

CARE CONSIDERATIONS FOR
HEALTHCARE WORKERS

There are many considerations for the healthcare worker caring for someone with MS. If you are a healthcare worker, the following issues are important for you to know and understand as you help your clients to achieve their highest state of functioning.

Remember that MS can be quite difficult and takes a lot of time to diagnose. Pay close attention to how clients describe their signs and symptoms. A good client history is important to an accurate diagnosis. Since it can take much time and effort to reach a diagnosis, the clients and their families can become frustrated and discouraged. Provide emotional support to both clients and families.

MS is a common problem, especially in North America. Be aware of risk factors that may make people more likely to develop MS. These include being a woman, having family members who have MS, living in certain climates (such as Northern Europe, North America, Australia, and New Zealand), eating a diet high in animal fats and dairy products, and having had certain viral infections.

Help your clients to learn about MS. They need to understand that there is no cure for this disease. They should know that there is no way to tell when signs and symptoms will appear or how severe they will be each time they come back. Your clients should be aware that most people do live productive lives for many years after being diagnosed with MS.

Although there is no single test that can definitely tell if a client has MS, there are several diagnostic tests that can provide helpful information. Be familiar with the tests and how clients need to prepare for them.

Treatment measures can lesson the severity of signs and symptoms and decrease the frequency of attacks of MS. Be aware of what medications your clients are taking. Find out about the side effects that can occur from these medications.

Most MS clients complain of extreme fatigue. Help your clients to understand that it is important to schedule rest periods throughout the day and to avoid extreme physical activity.

Help your clients understand the importance of living a healthy lifestyle. They should avoid stress and being exposed to infections as much as possible. They should eat a well-balanced

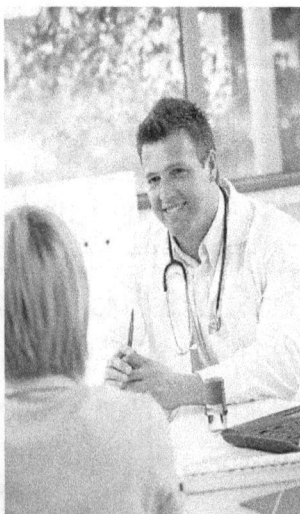

diet and consult their doctors about an exercise program that is right for them. They should work with healthcare professionals to learn new ways of performing activities of daily living. For persons with extreme fatigue and difficulty walking, the use of a cane, walker or wheelchair might be helpful. You may need to work with your clients to help them use such assistive devices safely.

Many MS clients have bowel and bladder problems. Help your clients to understand the treatment measures their doctors have prescribed. If medications are ordered, help your clients to learn how the drugs should be taken and what side effects may occur. Clients should eat a well-balanced diet with fruits and vegetables to help avoid constipation. Advise them to drink adequate fluids to help avoid bladder infections and constipation.

Encourage clients to seek help as needed for depression. Remember how important it is to provide emotional support to persons dealing with a chronic disease.

If your MS client lives at home, ensure that extra safety measures are in place. These may include keeping halls clutter-free, using slip-proof mats, keeping a light on at night, installing handrails, and wearing shoes with low heels. A microwave may be easier and safer to use than the stove for cooking. Clients should have an easy exit route out of the home. As well, they should have some way of calling for outside help if they need it.

It is safer for clients with MS to have a shower rather than a tub bath at home. Ensure your client uses a rubber mat on the floor of the shower. Advise showering when someone else is nearby. Your client may need to sit while showering. Advise your clients that soaking for a long time in a hot tub may increase muscle weakness.

Clients with MS should wear a MedicAlert or similar ID bracelet so that healthcare professionals will be aware of the condition should a medical emergency occur.

If clients are having sexual problems, be supportive and tactful. They may believe that nothing can help lessen such problems. Encourage them to seek help from the appropriate healthcare professionals.

Tell your clients that they must inform their doctors of ALL medications that they are taking. These include prescription drugs, over-the-counter drugs, herbal supplements, vitamins, weight loss products, and diet supplements. Some of these items may interfere with treatment measures prescribed by doctors to treat MS.

Clients who are especially bothered by heat and humidity will benefit from air conditioning in their home. If that is not an option, advise them to use a fan. Also, advise them to wear light clothing and drink plenty of cool drinks during hot weather.

Find out about the various health care organizations and/or support groups that might be able to offer information and support for persons with MS. Remind your clients that they should never use information from any organization, source, or Internet site unless they have discussed it with their doctor first! Some resources include:

MS Society of Canada
http://www.mssociety.ca

The National MS Society
http://www.nationalmssociety.org

The Mayo Clinic in the United States
http://www.mayoclinic.com

The National Institutes of Health
http://www.nih.gov

CONSIDER FOR A MOMENT ...

Is there an MS support group
in your area? If you are not sure,
find out. Inform your
clients about it.
They may want to join.

CASE EXAMPLE

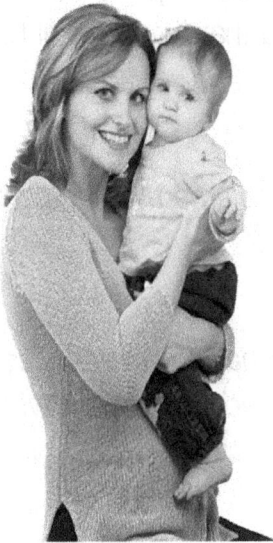

Your cousin, Melanie, is 30 years old and the mother of a ten-month old son. She and her family live in Chicago.

Melanie has been bothered by blurred vision and weakness in her legs for the past couple of years. These symptoms come and go but seem to get worse each time they return. The symptoms are particularly bad during hot, humid weather.

Melanie's symptoms returned several months ago, not long after the birth of her baby. They have not gone away. The blurred vision and leg weakness are worse now than they have ever been. Melanie also complains of being very tired, so tired that she "can hardly get out of bed in the morning." She is very nervous and worried.

You notice that her husband, Mark, is quite impatient with her. He accuses Melanie of over-reacting to her symptoms. He has told her that she could "get over it" if she tried.

Melanie has been told that she will have some tests done later this week. One of these tests is called magnetic resonance imaging (MRI). The test was explained to her. Melanie, however, forgot to ask if it would hurt. Now she is worried that the test will be painful.

What is it about Melanie's problems that indicate she may have MS?

Why do you think Melanie is having an MRI test done? Should she be concerned about pain with this procedure?

YOUR ANSWERS TO CASE EXAMPLE

SUGGESTED ANSWERS TO CASE EXAMPLE

What is it about Melanie's problems that indicate she may have MS?

Several factors, commonly found in persons with MS, are present in this case. Do you know what they are? If you said climate, sex, and age you're correct! The type of symptoms, the way they come and go, and the fact that they are worse in hot, humid weather should make you suspect MS too.

Mark does not seem very supportive. This might be causing Melanie added stress. She is also a new mother. Remember that stress and pregnancy have been linked with attacks of MS signs and symptoms.

Why do you think Melanie is having an MRI test done? Should she be concerned about pain with this procedure?

An MRI can help to diagnose many different conditions. It is also one of the best methods used to detect MS. This test may help Melanie's doctor to find out if she has the disease.

Melanie need not be concerned about pain. She should be told that there is generally no pain during an MRI procedure.

CONCLUSION

Multiple Sclerosis (MS) is a chronic disease that affects the brain and spinal cord. It usually, but not always, causes permanent disability. MS is a very common illness. It is particularly common in temperate climates. Canada has one of the highest rates of MS in the world.

The exact cause of MS is not known, although certain factors seem to make it more likely that someone will get the disease. Signs and symptoms of MS often come and go. It may take some time before a diagnosis can be made. Various tests are available to help with a diagnosis. Medications and other treatment measures help to slow down the disease progress or to manage the symptoms. Safety is an important issue in the care of people with this disease. Caregivers need to know about a variety of care considerations when working with people with MS.

Finally there has been a lot of media coverage for new hopeful treatment, as yet to be validated by the medical profession through clinical trials, involving neck-vein surgery for relieving congested veins, which in turn seems to help many MS sufferers. A vascular specialist Dr. Paolo Zamboni from Italy developed this and more information can be found on the internet.

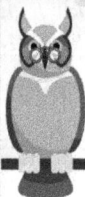

CHECK YOUR KNOWLEDGE

1. Describe the different types of MS.

2. What are the causes and risk factors for MS?

3. What are the signs and symptoms of MS?

4. Identify tests that can be done to help diagnose MS.

5. Describe treatment options for MS.

6. Discuss care considerations for healthcare workers assisting clients with MS.

TEST YOURSELF

Please circle to indicate the best answer:

1. Symptoms of MS may change from day to day and be difficult for the person to describe.

a. True

b. False

2. The first signs of MS may be vision problems or changes in sensation.

a. True

b. False

3. Research has shown that following a diet high in fruits and vegetables increases the risk of getting MS.

a. True

b. False

4. About 85% of those with MS have this type at the time they are diagnosed.

a. Benign

b. Relapsing-remitting

c. Primary progressive

d. Secondary progressive

5. Myelin is:

a. A type of drug used to treat MS.

b. A substance that covers and protects nerves.

c. A type of MS

d. A side effect of MS

6. To avoid constipation, you would encourage the person with MS to:

a. Eat foods high in fiber

b. Drink less water and other fluids

c. Drink fluids containing caffeine

d. Cut down on foods high in salt

7. The percentage of people with MS who continue to lead active, productive lives with the help of treatment is:

a. 10%

b. 30%

c. 50%

d. 70%

ANSWERS

1. a. True. Symptoms may change from day to day and be difficult for the person to describe.

2. a. True. In most people, vision problems or changes in sensation are the first signs that something might be wrong.

3. b. False. Research has shown that people at high risk for MS eat a diet high in animal fats and dairy products.

4. b. About 85% of persons with MS have the relapsing-remitting type at the time they are diagnosed.

5. b. Myelin is a substance that covers and protects the nerves in the central nervous system.

6. a. Adding fiber to the diet can help bowel problems such as incontinence and constipation.

7. d. About 70% of people with MS are able to continue to lead active, productive lives with the help of treatment.

REFERENCES

Bartelmo, J. (Ed). (2002). Handbook of medical-surgical nursing (3rd ed.). Springhouse, PA: Springhouse.

Eckman, M. and Priff, N. (1997). Diseases (2nd ed.). Springhouse, PA: Springhouse.

Health Talk. Intimacy and sexuality issues in women with MS. (2002). Retrieved March 23, 2002 from http://www.healthtalk. com

Holmes, H. N. (Ed.). (2000). Handbook of diseases, 2nd ed. Springhouse, PA: Springhouse.

Martin, N., Holt, N. B., & Hicks, D. (1981). Comprehensive rehabilitation nursing. New York: McGraw-Hill.

Mayoclinic.com (2002). Multiple sclerosis. What is MS? Retrieved August 19, 2002 from http://www.mayoclinic.com

Mayoclinic.com (2002). Multiple sclerosis. Self-care. Retrieved December 30, 2002 from http://www.mayoclinic.com/invoke. cfm?objectid=CEC491ED-C3B3-4B39-9E7473861360 32B4

Medline Plus Health Information. Associated Press, March 8, 2002. Serono says feds OK MS drug. Retrieved March 27, 2002 from http://www.nlm.nih.gov/medlineplus

National Institutes of Health. Adapted from a 1996 public domain publication from the Office of Scientific and Health Reports, National Institute of Neurological Disorders and Stroke. MS: Diagnosis & treatment/recent advances in research. Retrieved March 23, 2002 from http://www.telosnet.com/review/ms2. html

Pagana, K. D., & Pagana, T. J. (1999). Mosby's diagnostic and laboratory testmreference (4th ed.). St. Louis: Mosby.

Polman, C. H. (2000). Drug treatment of MS (Electronic version). British Medical Journal, August 19, 2000. Retrieved March 27, 2002 from http://www.findarticles.com

The Multiple Sclerosis Society of Canada (2002). MS information. Did you know ... Retrieved August 8, 2002 from http://www.mssociety.ca/en/information

The Multiple Sclerosis Society of Canada (2002). MS Information. Practical tips. Retrieved December 30, 2002 from http://www.mssociety.ca/en/information/tips.htm

Tran, M. (2001). MS (Electronic version). Gale Encyclopedia of Alternative Medicine, Retrieved March 23, 2002, from http://www.findarticles.com/cf_dls/g2603/0005/2603000536/print.jhml

www.ingramcontent.com/pod-product-compliance
Lightning Source LLC
Chambersburg PA
CBHW060655280326
41933CB00012B/2198